J.V. SINGH

The Ultimate Guide to Improving Your Vertical Jump

The guide for getting more explosive

Contents

1

Chapter 1: Understanding the Vertical Jump

Vertical jump is more than just leaping into the air. It reflects a combination of speed, strength, explosive power, and coordination. Understanding the mechanics, the physiology behind it, and its importance in sports performance is vital before diving into training routines and strength plans.

What is the Vertical Jump?

Vertical jump measures how high you can jump from a stationary standing position. It primarily assesses lower body power, leg strength, and coordination. A higher vertical jump indicates greater explosive strength, quickness, and the ability to generate force rapidly—skills that translate well to a variety of athletic activities.

Whether you are a basketball player aiming to dunk, a volleyball player looking for a powerful block, or simply a fitness enthusiast, improving your vertical jump will elevate your performance.

The Mechanics of a Vertical Jump

The movement of jumping involves coordinated action across multiple muscle groups. Understanding the mechanics behind your jump will help you identify areas of weakness, imbalances, or inefficient technique.

Here's a breakdown of the movement during a standard vertical jump:

1. Pre-Stretch (Preparation):The body shifts into a slight knee bend while the arms swing backward. This action stores elastic energy in the muscles.
2. Force Generation (Take-Off):The legs extend forcefully as the muscles contract. The quadriceps, glutes, hamstrings, calves, and core muscles work together to produce upward force.
3. Jump Execution:The explosive force propels the body upward. The arms swing forward during this phase, helping the body move efficiently toward the desired jump height.
4. Flight:During the air phase, the body maintains posture while maximizing the height gained.
5. Landing:The landing phase requires controlled strength to absorb the impact and stabilize the body, minimizing injury risk.

Muscles Involved in the Vertical Jump

Your jump relies on several muscle groups. Understanding these groups can help tailor workouts to strengthen them effectively:

Lower Body Muscles:

1. Quadriceps: These are located in the front of your thigh and are essential for knee extension during the take-off phase.
2. Glutes: The gluteus maximus is vital for explosive hip movement and generating upward force.
3. Calves (Gastrocnemius & Soleus): These muscles propel the body upward by extending the ankle rapidly during take-off.
4. Hamstrings: Located at the back of the legs, they work in conjunction with the quadriceps for knee movement and force transfer.

Core Muscles:

1. Abdominals: The abs stabilize the spine and support jumping movement.
2. Obliques: These aid in rotational stability and postural alignment during the jump.

The Importance of Explosive Power in Jumping

Explosive power is the foundation of jumping. Explosive power refers to the ability of your muscles to generate maximum force as quickly as possible. It relies on the rapid recruitment of fast-twitch muscle fibers, which are specialized for short bursts of power and speed.

Fast-twitch vs. Slow-twitch fibers:

1. Fast-twitch fibers: Specialized for quick, explosive actions

like sprinting and jumping. They produce large amounts of force in short durations.

2. Slow-twitch fibers: Designed for endurance rather than explosiveness and are more efficient at long-lasting, low-intensity activities.

Training with explosive movements increases the activation of fast-twitch fibers, allowing you to jump higher and react faster.

Why Your Vertical Jump Matters

The vertical jump isn't just a measure of athletic ability. It plays an integral role in performance across a variety of sports, including:

- Basketball: Essential for dunking and blocking shots.
- Volleyball: Key for spiking, blocking, and reaching for high serves.
- Track and Field: Important for jumping events like high jump, triple jump, and long jump.
- Fitness & General Health: A better vertical jump builds explosive strength, core stability, and overall physical conditioning.

Even outside of sports, improving your vertical jump can lead to better balance, improved coordination, and a reduction in the risk of injury.

Common Myths About the Vertical Jump

Many misconceptions surround the idea of improving vertical jump ability. Let's debunk some of the most common ones:

1. Myth 1: Only Genetics Matter.Genetics play a role, but vertical jump performance can absolutely be improved with proper training and consistency.
2. Myth 2: You Need to Jump Every Day.Overtraining can lead to injury. A proper balance of strength training, recovery, and practice is essential.
3. Myth 3: Strength Training Won't Help My Jump.Strength is a key part of improving jumping ability. Building leg and core strength provides the foundation for explosive movement.

Understanding the truth behind these myths will keep you focused on proper training rather than wasting time on ineffective strategies.

How Vertical Jump Relates to Other Performance Metrics

The vertical jump connects to other performance areas:

- Agility & Quickness: These are enhanced through power and explosiveness, translating into better reaction times.
- Balance: Improved core strength, facilitated by vertical jump training, enhances balance and coordination.
- Athleticism: Having a strong vertical jump showcases superior functional strength and power, which translates

to better performance across a variety of athletic activities.

Setting Your Goals

Before beginning your vertical jump improvement journey, take time to assess your current ability and set clear, measurable goals. Examples of goals could include:

- Increase your jump by X inches over a period of 3 months.
- Improve core stability to support explosive movements.
- Strengthen the glutes and hamstrings to improve take-off power.

Setting SMART (Specific, Measurable, Achievable, Relevant, Timely) goals will keep you motivated and on track.

Final Thoughts on Understanding Your Vertical Jump

Understanding the mechanics, purpose, and role of explosive power is your first step toward improving your jump. With knowledge in hand, you'll be better equipped to tailor your workouts, track your progress, and build a comprehensive training regimen.

2

Chapter 2: Getting Started with Vertical Jump Assessment

Before diving into the journey of improving your vertical jump, the first step is knowing your baseline. Assessing your current vertical jump will give you clarity about where you stand and how much progress you've made as you train. Chapter 2 will focus on methods for testing your vertical jump, understanding the results, and creating a roadmap for improvement based on those findings.

Why Assessment is Important

Assessments are a critical first step because they allow you to:

1. Determine Your Current Level: Knowing how high you can jump right now allows you to track progress.
2. Set Specific Goals: Whether you want to jump 6 inches higher or add 10 pounds of strength to your legs, assessments give you clear insights into what to target.
3. Identify Weaknesses: Assessments can highlight which

areas in your body might be underperforming. For example, your core might need more stability, or your glutes might require strengthening.

4. Track Progress: Regular testing allows you to measure the effectiveness of your training and ensure you're progressing toward your goals.

Without a baseline assessment, you would lack context for how far you've come or what specific training needs to be prioritized.

Common Methods to Assess Your Vertical Jump

There are several methods to measure your vertical jump. They range from simple tests using minimal equipment to more advanced testing protocols. Here are the most commonly used methods:

1. Standing Vertical Jump Test (Verbal or Visual)

This method is simple, accessible, and commonly used by athletes and coaches.

How to Perform the Standing Vertical Jump Test:

1. Stand next to a wall.
2. Reach your arm as high as possible and mark that point on the wall or use a measuring system like a vertec or a chalk mark.
3. Jump as high as you can vertically from a stationary standing position.
4. Mark the highest point you reach.

The difference between your standing reach and your jump reach gives you your vertical jump height.

2. The Vertec Device Test

The Vertec is an apparatus used by many sports performance experts to assess vertical jump. It consists of adjustable pegs that athletes attempt to touch at the peak of their jump.

Steps:

1. Record the highest peg you can reach before jumping.
2. Perform a maximal vertical jump and record the highest peg you can reach afterward.
3. Subtract the first measurement from the second to determine your vertical jump.

The Vertec method is precise and ensures consistency, making it ideal for coaches and professional athletes.

3. The Sargent Jump Test (Using Reach and Vertical Jump)

This test is a combination of standing reach and vertical jump measures and gives a good snapshot of an athlete's vertical jumping ability.

How to Perform the Sargent Jump Test:

1. Measure your standing reach.
2. Jump as high as you can and reach upward at the peak of your jump.
3. The difference between these two values provides your vertical jump ability.

This method gives insight into your explosive power and leaping capability.

4. Using Video Analysis for Assessment

With modern technology, you can use video analysis to assess your vertical jump. Simply film yourself jumping and analyze your body mechanics to spot weaknesses. Look for areas such as:

- Arm swing inefficiencies
- Poor knee bend during the jump
- Weak engagement of your glutes or hamstrings

Using slow-motion features in video editing software can make this analysis even more precise. Video analysis allows you to visualize and correct form flaws.

How to Interpret Your Results

Once you've completed your vertical jump test using one of the above methods, you'll have a numerical score. But what does this number mean? Here's how to interpret it:

Your individual goal depends on your sport and personal fitness journey. For instance:

- A basketball player may aim to reach a 28-inch vertical jump or more.
- A volleyball player may set a similar goal depending on blocking and spiking ability.

Understanding this scale allows you to set realistic, goal-oriented expectations.

Weaknesses & Strengths Assessment

While assessing the number is helpful, it's also critical to determine why your jump is at its current level. Here are some common areas to assess:

1. Leg Strength

The legs are responsible for most of the explosive power in a vertical jump. Weak glutes, hamstrings, and calves will result in poor jumping performance.

2. Core Stability

A weak core can affect your jumping mechanics. If you lack core stability, your entire jumping sequence will be less efficient.

3. Technique and Coordination

Even if you have good strength, improper technique can prevent you from reaching your full potential. Ensure your form is optimized for maximum efficiency.

4. Flexibility

Limited flexibility in the hips and hamstrings can hinder your ability to load and explode properly during a jump.

5. Explosive Power & Speed Training

Your ability to generate force quickly is vital. If you lack explosive power, plyometric training may help.

After testing and identifying areas of weakness, you can design a tailored program to improve your vertical jump effectively.

Next Steps: Setting Your Goals & Planning Your Training

Once you've assessed your vertical jump and determined areas of weakness, it's time to set goals and create a plan. Consider:

- Strength goals: Focusing on building strength in key muscle groups (glutes, quads, hamstrings).
- Plyometric goals: Adding explosive jumping exercises to your routine.
- Core training goals: Stabilizing your midsection for better posture and jump mechanics.

Your goals should follow the SMART system—Specific, Measurable, Achievable, Relevant, and Timely. Once you set these goals, you can move forward with a focused training regimen.

Final Thoughts: Knowledge is Power

The assessment is your starting point. Just like a roadmap helps you plan a journey, testing and assessments give you a clear path toward achieving your vertical jump goals. Understanding your starting point and the areas to improve will keep your workouts focused and goal-driven.

With all this knowledge in hand, you're ready to design a training program that builds strength, explosiveness, and skill.

3

Chapter 3: Strength & Conditioning for Jump Power

With your baseline assessment complete and an understanding of your current vertical jump abilities, the next logical step is to build a solid foundation. Strength and conditioning are essential components of any vertical jump training plan. The stronger your legs, core, and overall body, the higher you'll be able to jump.

In this chapter, we'll cover key aspects of strength training and conditioning exercises that directly contribute to explosive jumping ability. We'll examine the major muscle groups involved in vertical jumping, the science behind strength development, and a step-by-step approach to implementing effective workout routines.

Understanding the Role of Strength in Vertical Jump Performance

Before diving into workouts, let's break down why strength matters. A vertical jump is an explosive movement that relies heavily on the ability to generate force quickly. The muscles involved in this movement must be sufficiently developed to allow for the required explosive power.

The Major Muscle Groups Involved in a Vertical Jump

Your vertical jump relies on multiple muscle groups. Strengthening these groups will lead to improved jump height and overall performance:

1. Leg Muscles (Quads, Glutes, Hamstrings, and Calves):These muscles are directly responsible for propelling you off the ground during a jump. They act as the foundation for generating explosive power.

- Quadriceps (front of the thigh)
- Glutes (buttocks)
- Hamstrings (back of the thigh)
- Calves (gastrocnemius and soleus)

1. Core Muscles:The core stabilizes your body during takeoff and landing. A strong core improves posture, aids force transfer, and enhances overall athletic performance.

- Abdominals
- Obliques

- Lower back muscles

1. Hip Flexors:Hip flexors are involved in knee drive and proper movement mechanics during jumping. Strengthening them allows for better knee lift and fluid motion.
2. Arm Swing Contribution:While arms aren't a primary source of power, proper arm mechanics contribute to a more efficient jump. A well-timed arm swing helps coordinate your body movement during the jump.

Key Strength Training Principles for Vertical Jump Performance

Effective strength and conditioning for improving your vertical jump isn't just about lifting weights or training hard—it's about training smart. Here are the principles you'll need to follow:

1. Progressive Overload:To get stronger, you must progressively expose your muscles to greater stress. This means consistently increasing the amount of weight, repetitions, or intensity as you improve.
2. Explosive Training:Your training must include explosive movements. Strength work should focus on *power* by incorporating plyometrics and movements that mimic jumping.
3. Functional Strength:Train movements and patterns that mimic the demands of a vertical jump, such as squats, lunges, and plyometric exercises.
4. Recovery is Essential:Strength training places stress on your muscles and nervous system. Recovery time allows your body to repair and grow stronger. Incorporate rest

days and proper nutrition to support recovery.

5. Consistency and Frequency:You can't build strength overnight. Commit to regular, consistent workouts 3–4 days a week to see progress.

Strength & Conditioning Workout Plan

Now that you understand the science, let's put it into action. Below is a structured, sample strength and conditioning workout plan focused on improving your vertical jump by building strength and power in key areas.

Day 1: Lower Body Strength Training

This workout focuses on foundational leg strength—the primary driver of vertical jump performance.

1. Barbell Back Squats (4 x 6-8 reps)

- Muscles Worked: Glutes, quadriceps, hamstrings
- How to Perform:

1. Position the barbell across your shoulders and stand with feet shoulder-width apart.
2. Lower your body into a deep squat while keeping your back straight and chest up.
3. Push through your heels and return to a standing position.

2. Romanian Deadlifts (3 x 8-10 reps)

- Muscles Worked: Hamstrings, glutes, calves
- How to Perform:

1. Hold a barbell in front of you with your arms extended.
2. With a slight bend in the knees, hinge at the hips and lower the bar toward the ground.
3. Keep your back straight and push your hips forward to return to standing.

3. Calf Raises (4 x 15 reps)

- Muscles Worked: Calves
- How to Perform:

1. Stand on the edge of a step with your heels hanging off.
2. Rise onto the balls of your feet and lower back down in a controlled manner.

4. Hip Thrusts (3 x 8-10 reps)

- Muscles Worked: Glutes, hamstrings
- How to Perform:

1. Place a barbell or weight across your hips.
2. Press through your heels, thrust your hips upward, and then lower back down.

Day 2: Plyometric Training for Explosiveness

Plyometric exercises are critical for vertical jumping because they develop explosive strength.

1. Box Jumps (4 x 8 reps)

- How to Perform:

1. Start in a slight squat position with arms bent.
2. Explode upward, swinging your arms, and land softly on the box or platform.

2. Depth Jumps (3 x 8 reps)

- How to Perform:

1. Step off a low box, land, and immediately explode upward into a jump.

3. Broad Jumps (3 x 8 reps)

- How to Perform:

1. Start in an athletic stance.
2. Explosively jump forward as far as possible, landing softly.

Day 3: Core Stability & Recovery

Strong core muscles provide balance and transfer energy during jumps.

1. Plank Holds (3 x 30-60 seconds)

2. Russian Twists (3 x 15 reps per side)

3. Medicine Ball Slams (3 x 12 reps)

On this day, ensure you focus on mobility and recovery with stretching and foam rolling to maintain flexibility.

Progression and Periodization

The journey toward a better vertical jump requires progression and periodization. Periodization involves changing your workout variables (volume, intensity, or focus) over time to avoid plateaus and prevent injury.

- Weeks 1–4: Focus on building strength with compound movements like squats and deadlifts.
- Weeks 5–8: Shift the focus to explosive movements with plyometrics.
- Weeks 9–12: Combine strength and explosiveness into a hybrid plan.

Final Thoughts: Strength as the Foundation for Explosiveness

Strength isn't just about how much weight you can lift—it's about how efficiently your body uses that strength during explosive movements like jumping. Building the right kind of strength through compound lifts, plyometric training, and core stability will make all the difference in improving your vertical jump.

Stay consistent, listen to your body, and prioritize recovery. With dedication and the right approach, you'll soon see progress.

4

Chapter 4: Plyometric Training Techniques for Explosive Power

Having established a strong foundation with strength and conditioning, the next step is to incorporate explosive movements into your routine. Plyometric training focuses on developing fast-twitch muscle fibers, improving force production, and enhancing your body's ability to generate explosive power. This type of training is critical for achieving higher vertical jumps and improving athletic performance across a variety of sports.

In this chapter, we'll break down the most effective plyometric exercises, explore their benefits, and provide you with a sample workout plan to implement in your training routine.

Understanding Plyometric Training

Plyometric training involves quick, powerful movements that maximize the stretch-shortening cycle of your muscles. In simple terms, these exercises take your muscles through a rapid lengthening phase (eccentric) followed immediately by a rapid shortening phase (concentric), which generates explosive force.

Why Plyometrics Matter for Vertical Jump

Plyometric movements strengthen your neuromuscular system, improving your ability to jump by focusing on speed, power, and coordination. Incorporating these movements into your vertical jump program can lead to:

- Improved vertical jump height
- Increased explosiveness and agility
- Better coordination and overall athletic performance

For example, jumping onto a box, sprinting, or doing explosive squat jumps trains your muscles to exert maximum force quickly. This ability translates directly into better jumping performance.

Key Principles of Plyometric Training

Before we dive into the exercises, let's outline the key principles of effective plyometric training:

1. Focus on Quality Over Quantity:The goal is to perform explosive, powerful movements rather than simply completing a high number of repetitions. Always prioritize form and control during your training.
2. Adequate Rest Between Sets:Plyometric movements demand high energy and neuromuscular recovery. Avoid overtraining by allowing at least 1-2 minutes of rest between sets.
3. Progressive Overload:Like strength training, you should progressively increase the difficulty of your plyometric ex-

ercises over time by adding height, resistance, or intensity.

4. Consistency:Plyometric exercises require consistent training to develop neuromuscular adaptation. Aim to include these workouts 2-3 times per week.
5. Warm-Up Before Starting:Plyometric workouts are intense. Always warm up with dynamic stretches, light cardio, or mobility drills to prepare your muscles for explosive work.

Essential Plyometric Exercises for Vertical Jump

Below are some of the most effective plyometric exercises you can use to enhance your explosive power and vertical jump ability. These exercises target the legs, core, and coordination to build well-rounded jumping strength.

1. Box Jumps

One of the most well-known plyometric exercises, box jumps are great for improving explosive strength and coordination.

How to Perform Box Jumps:

1. Stand in front of a sturdy, elevated surface like a plyometric box or platform.
2. Begin in an athletic stance with your feet shoulder-width apart and arms slightly bent.
3. Swing your arms back, then forward, and use your legs to explode upward.
4. Land softly on top of the box, bending your knees slightly upon landing.
5. Step or jump back down and repeat for the desired number of repetitions.

Benefits:

- Builds leg explosiveness
- Enhances coordination and body control
- Improves landing mechanics

2. Depth Jumps

Depth jumps emphasize reactive strength and help improve your ability to jump quickly after landing.

How to Perform Depth Jumps:

1. Stand on a low box or step.
2. Step off the box and land softly on the ground.
3. As soon as you land, explode upward into a vertical jump.

Focus:

- Land with soft knees to reduce the risk of injury.
- Make the transition between landing and jumping as quick as possible.

Benefits:

- Improves reactive strength
- Trains fast-twitch muscle fibers
- Prepares your body for dynamic movements in sport or competition

3. Broad Jumps

Broad jumps help improve horizontal explosiveness and transfer strength into real-world movements like sprinting and jumping.

How to Perform Broad Jumps:

1. Start in an athletic stance with knees slightly bent.
2. Swing your arms and drive through your heels, jumping as far forward as possible.
3. Land softly and absorb the impact by bending your knees upon landing.

Repetitions:

- Complete 3-4 sets of 8-10 repetitions.

Benefits:

- Enhances jumping distance
- Builds core and leg strength
- Develops explosive power for athletic movements

4. Lateral Bounds

Lateral bounds are excellent for improving agility, lateral explosiveness, and single-leg power—key components for sports performance.

How to Perform Lateral Bounds:

1. Start in a slight squat position.
2. Jump sideways to the right, landing on your right foot.
3. Immediately jump back to the left, landing on your left foot.

Repetitions:

- Perform 3 sets of 8-10 repetitions each side.

Benefits:

- Builds lateral explosiveness
- Improves single-leg strength and balance
- Develops agility and coordination

5. Jump Squats

Jump squats combine strength and explosive movement to build lower body power.

How to Perform Jump Squats:

1. Begin in a standard squat position with your feet shoulder-width apart.
2. Explode upward as you extend your legs, jumping as high as you can.
3. Land softly and go straight into another squat.

Repetitions:

- Perform 3-4 sets of 10-12 repetitions.

Benefits:

- Strengthens your quads, glutes, and hamstrings
- Increases explosive power
- Improves jumping mechanics

Sample Plyometric Workout Routine

Here's a sample workout incorporating the plyometric exercises above. This workout is designed to improve explosive strength, reaction speed, and jumping ability.

Warm-Up (5-10 minutes)

- Light jog or dynamic stretches (arm circles, leg swings, high knees)

Workout Routine

1. Box Jumps: 4 x 8 reps
2. Depth Jumps: 3 x 8 reps
3. Broad Jumps: 3 x 10 reps
4. Lateral Bounds: 3 x 10 reps (each side)
5. Jump Squats: 4 x 10 reps

Cool Down

- Stretching focusing on calves, hamstrings, glutes, and quads.

Final Thoughts: Integrating Plyometrics into Your Plan

Plyometric training is a powerful way to bridge the gap between strength and explosive ability. Incorporate these exercises into your routine 2-3 times per week, focusing on quality over quantity. Remember, recovery is essential with plyometric work, as it places a lot of stress on your muscles and joints.

By combining strength and plyometric training, you'll build the foundation necessary to achieve peak vertical jump performance.

5

Chapter 5: Sport-Specific Training Drills

Now that you have a strong foundation in strength and plyometric training, the next logical step is to incorporate sport-specific drills into your training regimen. These drills not only improve your vertical jump but also integrate jumping mechanics into functional movement patterns. Sport-specific training ensures that your explosiveness, power, and agility are tailored toward your individual sport or athletic goals.

Whether you're a basketball player, volleyball player, soccer player, or sprinter, sport-specific drills will allow you to fine-tune your movement patterns, explosive power, and coordination. This chapter will outline various drills tailored for specific sports and how you can integrate them into your vertical jump program.

The Importance of Sport-Specific Training

Sport-specific training bridges the gap between general athleticism and the unique demands of particular sports. While strength and plyometric training build general power and explosiveness, sport-specific drills mimic the movement patterns, speed, and mechanics of your sport.

Why Sport-Specific Drills Matter:

1. Enhanced Skill Transfer:Sport-specific drills ensure that your training translates to actual competition scenarios. They simulate the movements you'll perform during games.
2. Improved Agility and Reaction Time:Many sports require quick changes of direction or reaction times. Sport-specific drills help develop these attributes while also improving your vertical jump.
3. Refinement of Technique:Training drills allow you to practice proper form and movement patterns under fatigue or pressure. This translates to better performance on the playing field or court.
4. Prevention of Injuries:Proper movement mechanics in sport-specific drills help reduce the risk of injury by teaching the body to move in efficient, natural ways.

With these principles in mind, let's break down some sport-specific drills you can use to elevate your vertical jump while enhancing your athletic performance.

Basketball Training Drills

Basketball demands explosive vertical jumps for dunking, blocking shots, and reaching for rebounds. Below are specific basketball drills you can incorporate into your vertical jump training:

1. Vertical Jump + Rebound Practice

This drill mimics the motion of jumping to grab a rebound in a real game.

How to Perform:

1. Start by standing in a basketball stance.
2. Explode upward, aiming for maximum vertical height.
3. Simulate catching a rebound by extending your arms upon reaching your peak jump height.
4. Land softly and return to a defensive stance.
5. Repeat for 3 sets of 8-10 reps.

2. Ladder Drills + Vertical Jump

Agility is vital in basketball. Combine ladder footwork drills with a vertical jump to enhance agility and explosiveness.

How to Perform:

1. Set up an agility ladder on the ground.
2. Perform quick footwork patterns through the ladder (e.g., two-footed hops, lateral shuffling).
3. At the end of the ladder, perform an explosive vertical jump.

Repeat for 3-4 rounds, focusing on explosive movement and footwork.

Volleyball Training Drills

Volleyball players rely on explosive vertical jumps for blocking, spiking, and jumping to reach balls. These drills will mimic the explosive power needed for those movements.

1. Block Jump Practice

This drill is specific to volleyball blocking mechanics.

How to Perform:

1. Start in a volleyball stance near a wall or net.
2. Jump explosively, reaching your arms overhead as if blocking a spike.
3. Land softly and return to your starting position.

Repetitions:

Complete 3 sets of 10-12 repetitions.
Soccer Training Drills
While soccer isn't a sport directly focused on vertical jumping, soccer players benefit from explosive speed and aerial jumping ability during headers and sprinting.

1. Jump & Sprint Drill

How to Perform:

1. Start in an athletic position near a marker or sprint line.
2. Explode upward into a vertical jump as you initiate the sprint.
3. Land and transition into a sprint, covering a short distance.

Repeat this sequence 6-8 times.

Football/Sprinting Training Drills

Football requires agility, quickness, and explosive speed. For football players, vertical jumping is essential for catching passes, tackling, and blocking.

1. Sprint + Vertical Jump Drill

How to Perform:

1. Sprint for 10 yards.
2. Jump as explosively as possible at the end of the sprint.
3. Land softly and recover.

Repeat for 4-5 rounds.

Integrating Sport-Specific Drills into Your Training Plan

Now that you have some sport-specific drills, you may wonder how to integrate them into your weekly training routine.

Sample Weekly Sport-Specific Vertical Jump Training Plan:

Adjust these sessions based on your sport and your personal recovery needs. The idea is to maintain balance between explosive vertical jump work, sport skills, and recovery to prevent overtraining.

Final Thoughts: Building Sport-Specific Consistency

Integrating sport-specific drills into your routine allows you to fine-tune your explosive strength and jumping mechanics in the context of your unique sport. While strength and plyometric work are vital for building a foundation, the ability to translate that power into sport-specific movements sets the elite athletes apart.

Consistency is key. Just as you would strengthen your legs or core with plyometric exercises, sport-specific drills should be trained regularly—aim for 2-3 times per week depending on your sport and personal recovery ability.

6

Chapter 6: Recovery Methods and Injury Prevention

Training to improve your vertical jump and athletic performance isn't just about rigorous workouts and explosive movements. Recovery plays just as vital a role in the process as the training itself. Recovery ensures that your muscles repair, your body adapts, and your nervous system stays primed for the next training session or competition. Without proper recovery strategies, overtraining and injury can derail your progress and limit your performance.

In this chapter, we'll explore effective recovery strategies, techniques for injury prevention, and how to balance rest and training for optimal progress.

The Importance of Recovery

Recovery isn't simply about taking a break from training; it's a systematic approach that allows the body time to repair and rebuild. When you perform strength and plyometric training or sport-specific drills, microscopic tears occur in your muscles.

Recovery provides time for these muscles to rebuild stronger and more efficient than before.

Why Recovery Matters:

1. Muscle Repair and Growth:Exercise creates stress on your muscles, and recovery allows them to repair and grow stronger.
2. Prevention of Injury:Overtraining without adequate rest can lead to injuries, such as tendonitis, sprains, or muscle strains. Recovery reduces these risks.
3. Restores Energy Levels:Intense training depletes glycogen stores. Recovery allows your body to replenish these energy reserves.
4. Mental Health Benefits:Taking breaks prevents mental burnout. Training every day without rest can lead to mental fatigue and decreased motivation.
5. Adaptation to Training:Recovery periods allow your body to adapt to the new physical demands you place on it, improving your overall performance.

Effective Recovery Strategies

Recovery can take many forms. Below are several recovery techniques that, when used consistently, will ensure you're prepared for the next training session.

1. Sleep – The Foundation of Recovery

Sleep is the most important recovery tool. It's during sleep that the body performs the most significant repair and restoration. Aim for 7-9 hours of quality sleep each night to optimize recovery.

How Sleep Helps Recovery:

- Muscle Repair: Growth hormone is released during deep sleep, which aids in tissue repair and growth.
- Central Nervous System Restoration: Your nervous system needs sleep to recover from the stress of training.
- Replenishment of Energy Stores: Sleep restores glycogen levels, ensuring energy for the next workout.

Tips for Better Sleep:

1. Establish a regular sleep schedule (go to bed and wake up at the same time each day).
2. Avoid screens (phone, laptop, TV) at least one hour before bedtime, as blue light can interfere with melatonin production.
3. Ensure your bedroom is cool, quiet, and dark for optimal sleep conditions.
4. Practice relaxation techniques such as meditation or reading to unwind before bed.

2. Active Recovery – Keeping Movement Low-Impact

Active recovery involves light, low-impact movement on rest days to promote blood flow and aid muscle repair without overtaxing your system. Active recovery allows your body to flush out lactic acid and other byproducts that accumulate during intense exercise.

Examples of Active Recovery:

- Walking or Hiking: Gentle walking outdoors or on a treadmill.
- Swimming or Cycling: Low-impact, aerobic exercises.
- Yoga or Stretching: Improves flexibility and enhances mobility.
- Foam Rolling: Relieves tension and promotes circulation.

When to Use Active Recovery:

Incorporate these activities on rest days or between intense training sessions. They're especially beneficial for preventing soreness and maintaining range of motion.

3. Nutrition – Fueling Recovery from the Inside Out

Recovery isn't just about rest; it's also about nutrition. The food you eat has a direct impact on how quickly your body repairs and rebuilds.

Key Nutritional Principles for Recovery:

1. Protein:Protein is vital for muscle repair and growth. Aim for 0.7-1 gram of protein per pound of body weight daily, sourced from lean meats, fish, dairy, or plant-based options.
2. Carbohydrates:Carbs replenish glycogen stores that are depleted during workouts. Opt for complex carbohydrates like sweet potatoes, brown rice, oats, and whole-grain bread.
3. Healthy Fats:Fats are important for hormone production and overall energy levels. Incorporate sources like avocados, nuts, seeds, and olive oil.
4. Hydration:Staying hydrated is vital for overall health and recovery. Aim to drink at least 2-3 liters of water daily, more if you sweat a lot during training.

Sample Post-Workout Meal:

- Grilled chicken with quinoa and steamed broccoli.
- Sweet potato with black beans and avocado.
- Protein smoothie with berries, spinach, and protein powder.

4. Stretching and Flexibility

Stretching is an often-overlooked part of recovery, but it can help maintain mobility, reduce soreness, and prevent injuries. Stretching should be performed post-workout when your muscles are warm.

Types of Stretching:

1. Static Stretching: Hold each stretch for 20-30 seconds. Examples include seated hamstring stretches, quad stretches, and calf stretches.
2. Dynamic Stretching: Gentle, controlled movements to prepare the body for movement or sport. Examples include leg swings, arm circles, and hip rotations.

Make stretching a habit after every workout, particularly focusing on areas that feel tight.

5. Foam Rolling and Myofascial Release

Foam rolling is a form of self-myofascial release that improves blood flow, breaks up muscle adhesions, and enhances recovery.

How to Use a Foam Roller:

1. Place the foam roller on the targeted muscle group (e.g., quads, calves, hamstrings).
2. Slowly roll back and forth over the area for 30-60 seconds.
3. Pause at tight or sore spots to allow the muscle to release tension.

Foam rolling should be used post-workout or on rest days to encourage muscle recovery.

Injury Prevention Strategies

Preventing injuries is a crucial part of recovery. Many injuries can be prevented by incorporating proper techniques, warming up, stretching, and managing training volume.

1. Warm-Up and Cool Down:

Always spend 5-10 minutes warming up before your workout to prepare your body for intense exercise. Similarly, cool down after training by stretching and gradually reducing your heart rate.

2. Strengthen Your Weak Areas:

Identify imbalances or weak points in your body and incorporate strength exercises to address them.

3. Listen to Your Body:

If you're feeling pain, fatigue, or discomfort, stop the activity and rest. Overtraining can lead to chronic injuries over time.

Balancing Training and Recovery

Finding the right balance between training and recovery is essential. Overtraining can hinder your progress and put you at risk for injury, while too much rest can reduce your athletic performance.

Tips for Balancing Recovery and Training:

1. Plan rest days strategically into your weekly workout schedule.
2. Use periodization—a structured plan that cycles through high-intensity and recovery periods.
3. Monitor your body's signs of overtraining (persistent

soreness, irritability, difficulty sleeping, or decreased performance).

Final Thoughts on Recovery

Recovery is the unsung hero of any successful training regimen. It ensures that your body remains healthy, strong, and capable of performing at its best. By incorporating sleep, proper nutrition, active recovery, stretching, and mindfulness into your routine, you'll set yourself up for long-term success in building a higher vertical jump and excelling in your sport

7

Chapter 7: Programming Your Vertical Jump Plan

Creating a structured workout plan is critical for maximizing your vertical jump progress. You've learned the advanced techniques and their individual benefits, but without proper programming, you might not see the results you're aiming for. Programming ensures that your workouts are purposeful, balanced, and allow for recovery while progressing over time.

This chapter will teach you how to structure your training week, plan periodization, create balanced routines, and stay on track toward achieving your vertical jump goals.

Understanding Periodization in Vertical Jump Training

Before diving into workout programming, it's important to understand the concept of periodization. Periodization is a systematic approach to training that breaks your workout plan into distinct phases. These phases emphasize different goals and allow your body to recover, adapt, and improve over time without plateauing or overtraining.

Types of Periodization to Consider:

1. Linear Periodization:

- This approach involves gradually increasing the intensity and volume of your workouts over time. You may focus on strength building in the initial phase and transition into explosive power in later stages.

1. Undulating Periodization:

- This strategy involves regularly changing intensity and volume from week to week. For example, one week might focus on heavy strength training, while the next emphasizes explosive power with plyometric drills.

1. Block Periodization:

- Workouts are broken into distinct "blocks" focusing on specific skills or aspects of fitness, such as strength, explosiveness, or conditioning.

Understanding how to strategically structure these phases can help you avoid burnout while continually making progress toward your goal.

How to Structure Your Weekly Training Program

Your weekly workout schedule should balance strength training, plyometrics, sprint drills, recovery, and mobility work. Below is an example of how to structure a weekly training plan that focuses on progressive overload while incorporating recovery and all aspects of vertical jump training:

Sample Weekly Vertical Jump Training Plan

Day 1: Lower Body Strength Day

Focus on foundational strength to build the foundation for explosive movements.

Exercises:

1. Barbell Squats - 4 sets of 6-8 reps
2. Romanian Deadlifts - 3 sets of 8-10 reps
3. Walking Lunges - 3 sets of 10 reps each leg
4. Leg Press - 4 sets of 8 reps
5. Calf Raises - 4 sets of 12-15 reps

Key Focus: Strengthen the glutes, quads, hamstrings, and calves to improve your jumping power.

Day 2: Plyometric Power Day

Train your explosive power with a focus on explosive movement patterns.

Exercises:

1. Depth Jumps - 4 sets of 5-6 reps
2. Broad Jumps - 4 sets of 6-8 reps
3. Single-Leg Box Jumps - 3 sets of 6 reps per leg
4. Lateral Hurdle Hops - 3 sets of 8 reps per side
5. Sprint Intervals - 8 x 20-meter sprints with active recovery in between.

Key Focus: Improve your reactive strength and neuromuscular coordination.

Day 3: Core & Stability Work

A strong core is critical for maintaining stability and generating force during explosive movements.

Exercises:

1. Plank Holds - 3 sets of 60 seconds
2. Russian Twists (with or without medicine ball) - 4 sets of 12 reps per side
3. Hanging Leg Raises - 3 sets of 10-12 reps
4. Cable Woodchoppers - 3 sets of 10 reps per side
5. Stability Ball Rollouts - 3 sets of 10-12 reps

Key Focus: Enhance core strength, stability, and injury prevention.

Day 4: Recovery and Mobility

Rest is an essential part of any well-designed workout program. This day focuses on active recovery to promote blood flow, flexibility, and mobility.

Recovery Activities:

1. Yoga or stretching routines for full-body flexibility
2. Foam rolling and mobility drills for recovery and injury prevention
3. Light cycling or swimming for 30-45 minutes to stay active without overstressing the body

Day 5: Sprint & Agility Day

Combine speed, agility, and conditioning into one explosive day.

Sprint Workouts:

1. 20-meter sprints x 10 reps
2. 40-meter sprints x 6 reps
3. Resisted Sprints (using sleds or hills) - 6 x 20 meters

Agility Workouts:

1. Ladder drills (in-and-out lateral movement) - 3 sets of 10 repetitions
2. Cone drills with rapid changes of direction - 4 sets of 8 reps each.

Key Focus: Train your quickness, acceleration, and change-of-direction ability.

Day 6: Full-Body Strength & Jump Work

Combine your strength-building principles with explosive jump training.
Strength Exercises:

1. Deadlifts - 4 sets of 5 reps
2. Barbell Hip Thrusts - 4 sets of 8 reps
3. Bulgarian Split Squats - 4 sets of 10 reps each leg

Jump & Explosive Work:

1. Medicine Ball Slams - 4 sets of 8 reps
2. Lateral Box Jumps - 4 sets of 6 reps
3. Overhead Medicine Ball Throws - 3 sets of 8 reps

Key Focus: Build strength while also focusing on dynamic movement patterns and explosive power.

Day 7: Recovery & Active Rest

This day is for light movement to promote recovery and mental preparation for the next week of training.
Recovery Options:

- Gentle walking, swimming, or cycling for 30 minutes
- Light stretching or yoga
- Engage in light mobility and breathing work

How to Progress in Your Vertical Jump Training

Progressive Overload:

To see improvement over time, ensure that you're implementing progressive overload. This means gradually increasing the intensity, volume, or complexity of your workouts.
Examples include:

- Adding weight to strength exercises.
- Increasing the number of sets/reps over time.
- Increasing sprint distances or depth jump intensity.

Tracking Your Progress:

Always track your lifts, sets, and the number of reps you perform. This helps you identify when to increase intensity, when you're improving, or if you need to adjust recovery.

Listen to Your Body:

Avoid overtraining by paying attention to your body's signals. If you notice fatigue, soreness, or drops in performance, incorporate an extra recovery day.

Conclusion

Creating a well-structured program with strategic periodization and clear goals is the cornerstone of improving your vertical jump. This plan balances strength, plyometric training, sprint drills, recovery, and mental focus to ensure long-term progress and prevent burnout.

8

Chapter 8: Nutrition & Recovery Strategies to Maximize Your Results

You've now learned how to create and execute an effective vertical jump training program. But even the best training plan can fall short without proper nutrition and recovery. Your body is like a machine; just as a car needs fuel and regular maintenance to function properly, your body requires the right nutrients, rest, and recovery strategies to perform at its best.

This chapter will outline the importance of nutrition and recovery, how they directly affect your performance, and provide actionable strategies to ensure your body is primed for progress.

Why Nutrition Matters for Vertical Jump Training

Nutrition is the foundation upon which your body can build strength, repair muscles, and recover from intense workouts. The food you eat provides the energy to power through explosive movements, the building blocks to strengthen your muscles, and the tools to maintain hormonal balance and recovery.

Here's how nutrition supports vertical jump goals:

1. Energy: Carbohydrates are your body's primary energy source. They fuel your workouts and sprint drills. Without them, you'll struggle to maintain intensity.
2. Muscle Repair & Growth: Protein is essential for repairing muscle tissue and building new muscle after intense training. This is crucial for strength and explosive power.
3. Hydration: Staying hydrated ensures optimal performance during training and prevents fatigue and injury.
4. Recovery: Healthy fats, micronutrients, and proper rest work synergistically to repair damaged cells and reduce inflammation.

Building Your Nutrition Plan

To fuel your vertical jump training effectively, prioritize a diet that is balanced, nutrient-rich, and aligned with your goals. Your meals should focus on carbohydrates, proteins, healthy fats, and hydration.

Macronutrients for Vertical Jump Success

Here's the breakdown of macronutrients and their role in your vertical jump journey:

1. Carbohydrates (Energy Source)

Carbohydrates are vital for maintaining energy during high-intensity workouts. They are stored in your muscles as glycogen, which powers sprinting, explosive jumping, and other training movements.

Sources of Carbohydrates:

- Whole grains (brown rice, oats, quinoa, whole wheat bread)
- Sweet potatoes
- Fruits (bananas, apples, berries)
- Vegetables (spinach, carrots, broccoli)

Tip: Aim to eat complex carbohydrates before workouts to provide sustained energy.

2. Protein (Repair & Growth)

Protein is essential for repairing muscle tissue after exercise. A post-workout protein intake ensures your body can rebuild and grow stronger.

Sources of Protein:

- Chicken, turkey, lean beef
- Fish (salmon, tuna, tilapia)
- Eggs
- Dairy (milk, yogurt, cheese)
- Plant-based proteins (lentils, beans, chickpeas, tofu)

Recommended Intake: Aim for 1.2 to 2 grams of protein per kilogram of body weight daily, depending on your activity levels.

3. Healthy Fats (Reduce Inflammation & Hormonal Support)

Healthy fats support recovery by reducing inflammation, enhancing joint health, and balancing hormones.
Sources of Healthy Fats:

- Avocados
- Nuts and seeds (almonds, chia seeds, walnuts)
- Olive oil
- Fatty fish like salmon

4. Hydration

Water is essential for all bodily functions, from energy metabolism to temperature regulation. Dehydration can impair performance, cause fatigue, and hinder recovery.
Hydration Guidelines:

- Drink half your body weight in ounces of water daily. For example, a 150-pound person should aim for around 75 ounces of water.
- During intense workouts, replenish lost fluids by drinking water every 15-30 minutes.

Supplements to Consider

While the focus should always be on whole, nutrient-rich foods, supplements can help fill gaps and support specific goals.

Creatine Monohydrate

Creatine has been shown to improve strength, speed, and power, making it a useful addition to a vertical jump training program.

Protein Powder

If you struggle to meet your protein intake goals with food alone, whey or plant-based protein powders can provide a convenient and fast-digesting protein source post-workout.

BCAAs (Branched-Chain Amino Acids)

These essential amino acids can help reduce muscle breakdown during workouts and support recovery.

Note: Always consult a healthcare professional before incorporating new supplements into your routine.

Timing Your Nutrition

Eating at the right time can make a huge difference in performance and recovery. Here are some key windows to prioritize:

Pre-Workout:

Your pre-workout meal should include complex carbohydrates and a moderate amount of protein. Avoid heavy or fatty foods right before training to prevent discomfort.

Example Pre-Workout Meals:

- Oatmeal with banana and almond butter
- Grilled chicken, sweet potato, and steamed broccoli
- Whole wheat toast with scrambled eggs

Post-Workout:

Post-workout meals are essential for muscle repair and recovery. Aim for a mix of carbohydrates and protein within 30 minutes to 2 hours after a workout.

Example Post-Workout Meals:

- Grilled fish with quinoa and steamed vegetables
- Protein shake with berries and a scoop of whey protein
- Turkey sandwich on whole-grain bread with a side of fruit

Throughout the Day:

Consistency matters. Maintain a steady intake of water, healthy fats, and balanced snacks to ensure recovery and maintain energy levels.

Hydration Reminder: Every time you feel thirsty, drink water. Proper hydration should become a daily habit.

The Role of Sleep & Recovery

Training hard is only one side of the coin. Recovery is just as important, if not more so, in improving your performance and reducing the risk of injury. Your body needs time to repair, grow, and adapt after intense training sessions.

Sleep: Your Body's Recovery Tool

Sleep is essential for hormone production (especially growth hormone) and muscle repair. Aim for 7-9 hours of quality sleep each night to give your body enough time to recover.

Rest Days:

Active rest can be as effective as complete rest. Use these days for light stretching, walking, yoga, or foam rolling to maintain blood flow and flexibility.

Active Recovery Techniques:

- Yoga and stretching routines
- Swimming or cycling at low intensity
- Foam rolling to reduce muscle tension and soreness

Conclusion

Your training will only be as effective as your recovery and nutrition. Proper nutrition, hydration, and sleep fuel your workouts, repair your muscles, and optimize your body for growth. Implement these strategies alongside your vertical jump program, and you'll set yourself up for greater success.

By prioritizing both recovery and nutrition, you'll build a strong foundation that will complement all the explosive training you're putting in.

9

Chapter 9: Mental Strategies and Visualization for Peak Performance

Your body is now equipped with the training and recovery methods to improve your vertical jump, but have you considered the power of your mind? Your mental state is just as critical as your physical fitness when it comes to achieving success in sports and vertical jump training. Mental preparation can influence your ability to push through challenges, stay focused, and unlock your full potential.

This chapter will explore various mental strategies, visualization techniques, goal-setting methods, and mindset shifts to help you break through mental barriers and maintain peak performance on and off the court or field.

The Power of Mental Strength

When training for a goal as ambitious as improving your vertical jump, it's easy to hit mental roadblocks. These can include feelings of doubt, frustration with slow progress, or just a lack of motivation during tough workouts. Developing mental strength is about learning how to control these emotions, stay disciplined, and focus on your "why."

Why Mental Strength Matters

Your mental game determines how you handle pressure, recover from setbacks, and push through intense physical challenges. When you build mental toughness, you are better prepared to:

1. Overcome fear and self-doubt.
2. Push through physical discomfort during tough workouts.
3. Develop consistency even on days when motivation is low.
4. Visualize and manifest successful outcomes.

Think of mental strength as the bridge between your physical fitness and your performance.

Visualization: Seeing Your Success

Visualization is a powerful mental tool that athletes, coaches, and top performers have used for decades. It involves mentally rehearsing a skill, movement, or goal as though you're actually performing it. Your mind and body respond to imagined experiences almost as vividly as actual ones.

How Visualization Works

Research shows that visualization engages the same neural pathways in your brain as physical practice. When you mentally practice an action (e.g., jumping for a dunk or reaching a box in a vertical jump), your body begins to prepare for the movement, and your performance improves.

Types of Visualization

There are a few different ways to use visualization in your vertical jump training:

1. Mental Rehearsal: Visualize yourself performing the perfect jump, from the moment of preparation to the explosive leap and landing.
2. Successful Outcome Visualization: Picture yourself clearing a new height or achieving a vertical jump goal, such as dunking or completing a box jump.
3. Scenario Visualization: Imagine yourself in a high-pressure moment during competition and rehearse how you would successfully execute your jump.

How to Incorporate Visualization

The key to effective visualization is to make it as vivid and realistic as possible. Here's how you can integrate it into your training:

1. Set the Scene:

Close your eyes and picture your environment. Visualize the gym, the track, or the basketball court as you perform the jump.

2. Focus on Details:

Pay attention to every detail—how your muscles engage, how your body feels as you jump, and the motion of your limbs.

3. Use All Senses:

Engage your senses during visualization. Think about the sound of your feet on the ground, the tension in your muscles, and the sight of your hands reaching toward the basket.

4. Repeat Often:

Visualization works best when you make it a consistent part of your routine. Spend 5-10 minutes each day visualizing your goal or performance.

Visualization Example: Perfecting the Vertical Jump

1. Start by Imagining Your Preparation:Picture yourself standing at the starting position for your jump. Focus on your breathing, posture, and mindset.
2. Visualize the Explosive Movement:See yourself bending your knees, swinging your arms, and launching upward with maximum force.
3. Visualize the Apex of the Jump:Imagine reaching your peak height, your arms extended, and your body soaring through the air.
4. Envision the Landing:Picture yourself landing smoothly with balance, stability, and confidence.

When you mentally visualize every step in detail, you create a blueprint for your body to follow during actual physical performance.

Goal Setting: The Foundation of Success

Mental strategies are most effective when paired with clear, well-defined goals. Your goals act as a road map, providing direction and motivation throughout your journey. They give your training meaning and ensure you stay on track, even when obstacles arise.

Setting SMART Goals

The SMART acronym is a tried-and-true method for setting clear, achievable goals:

- Specific: Your goal should be clear and well-defined.
- Measurable: You should be able to track your progress.
- Achievable: The goal should challenge you but still be realistic.
- Relevant: The goal should align with your overall vertical jump aspirations.
- Time-bound: Set a deadline to give your goal urgency and focus.

Examples of SMART Goals for Vertical Jump Training:

1. Short-Term Goal:"I will improve my vertical jump by 3 inches in the next 4 weeks by completing my workout plan consistently."
2. Medium-Term Goal:"I will achieve a 30-inch vertical jump within the next 6 months by incorporating strength, plyometrics, and recovery strategies into my training."
3. Long-Term Goal:"I will be able to dunk a basketball during

a game by the end of the year."

By setting clear, incremental goals, you set yourself up for success while maintaining motivation.

Developing a Growth Mindset

A growth mindset is the belief that your abilities, skills, and performance can be improved through effort, persistence, and dedication. This mindset empowers athletes to embrace challenges and learn from mistakes.

Fixed Mindset vs. Growth Mindset

- Fixed Mindset: Believing that your abilities are static and that you can't improve past a certain point.
- Growth Mindset: Believing that you can improve with consistent effort, practice, and learning.

How to Cultivate a Growth Mindset

1. Embrace Challenges: See challenges as opportunities to grow rather than as threats.
2. Learn from Setbacks: Instead of viewing failures as defeats, treat them as lessons and opportunities for improvement.
3. Celebrate Progress: Acknowledge every small victory along your journey. Each step forward builds confidence.
4. Focus on Effort: The effort you put into your workouts is just as important as the results.

When you adopt a growth mindset, you begin to see training and challenges as exciting opportunities rather than barriers.

Building Confidence

Confidence is a mental edge that allows you to believe in your ability to perform under pressure. Just like physical strength, confidence can be built through preparation, repetition, and mindset.

Ways to Build Confidence:

1. Track Your Progress: Seeing how far you've come can boost your motivation and belief in your abilities.
2. Positive Self-Talk: Replace negative thoughts with positive affirmations. For example, "I can do this" or "I am improving every day."
3. Visualize Success: As previously mentioned, visualization creates a mental blueprint for success and builds confidence.

Confidence isn't just about feeling good; it's about trusting that you've done the work to succeed.

10

Conclusion

Your journey to improving your vertical jump isn't just about physical strength or recovery—it's also about mental preparation. By implementing visualization, goal setting, and mental strategies, you create a mindset that complements your physical training. Mental strategies are the key to unlocking your potential and achieving the explosive power you're striving for.

Now that you have the mental tools and strategies in your arsenal, you're prepared to move confidently into the next phase of your training journey.

Conclusion

Improving your vertical jump is a holistic journey that combines strength, mobility, recovery, and mental preparation. By mastering the physical and mental tools outlined in this guide, you can push through self-doubt, setbacks, and challenges to achieve peak performance. Consistency, discipline, and the right mindset are your greatest allies in this journey. Remember, progress isn't always linear, but with the tools and strategies you've learned here, you're well-equipped to tackle obstacles and stay the course.

As you embark on this journey, it's essential to remember that success is not solely defined by the height you achieve. The process of improving your vertical jump is just as important as the outcome. Every workout, every rep, and every visualization session brings you closer to your goal. The journey is where the real growth happens, and it's where you'll develop the mental and physical strength to overcome any obstacle.

Don't be discouraged by setbacks or plateaus. They are an inevitable part of the journey, and they provide an opportunity to reassess, adjust, and come back stronger. Stay focused on your goals, and remind yourself why you started this journey in the first place. Whether it's to improve your athletic performance, enhance your overall fitness, or simply to challenge yourself, your "why" is what will drive you to succeed.

As you progress, you'll notice changes not just in your physical abilities but also in your mental toughness and confidence. You'll develop a growth mindset, learning to embrace challenges and view failures as opportunities for growth. You'll become more resilient, more focused, and more determined.

The journey to improving your vertical jump is not just about physical training; it's about mental preparation, nutrition, recovery, and consistency. It's about developing a holistic approach to fitness that encompasses every aspect of your being. By committing to this journey, you're not just improving your vertical jump; you're transforming your entire self.

So, stay committed, stay focused, and trust the process. Believe in yourself, and never stop growing. With dedication, hard work, and the right mindset, you'll achieve your goals and unlock your full potential. The sky's the limit, and with the tools and strategies outlined in this guide, you're ready to take your vertical jump to new heights.

Thank You for reading and investing your time into this book and if you thought this book was helpful and insightful i would be extremely grateful if u can leave a review on this book.

References

Baker, D., & Nance, S. (1999). The relation between strength and power in professional rugby league players. *Journal of Strength and Conditioning Research, 13*(3), 224–229. https://doi.org/10.1519/00124278-199908000-00010

Bobbert, M. F., & van Ingen Schenau, G. J. (1988). Coordination in vertical jumping. *Journal of Biomechanics, 21*(3), 249–262. https://doi.org/10.1016/0021-9290(88)90175-3

Bompa, T. O., & Buzzichelli, C. (2018). *Periodization: Theory and methodology of training* (6th ed.). Human Kinetics.

Cissik, J. (2014). *Plyometric exercises with weights.* Human Kinetics.

Comfort, P., Bullock, N., & Pearson, S. J. (2012). A comparison of strength and power characteristics between players from professional and amateur rugby league. *Journal of Strength and Conditioning Research, 26*(10), 2688–2694. https://doi.org/10.1519/JSC.0b013e318241382a

Komi, P. V. (Ed.). (2008). *Strength and power in sport* (2nd ed.). Blackwell Science Ltd.

Newton, R. U., & Kraemer, W. J. (1994). Developing explosive muscular power: Implications for a mixed methods training strategy. *Strength and Conditioning Journal, 16*(5), 20–31. https://doi.org/10.1519/1073-6840(1994)016<0020:DEMP>2.3.CO;2

Rippetoe, M., & Kilgore, L. (2005). *Starting strength: Basic barbell training.* Aasgaard Company.

Schmidtbleicher, D. (1992). Training for power events. In P. V. Komi (Ed.), *Strength and power in sport* (pp. 381–395). Blackwell Scientific.

Sheppard, J. M., & Young, W. B. (2006). Agility literature review: Classifications, training, and testing. *Journal of Sports Sciences, 24*(9), 919–932. https://doi.org/10.1080/02640410500457109

Spooner Physical Therapy. (n.d.). *10 exercises to improve your vertical jump.* Retrieved December 8, 2024, from https://www.spoonerpt.com/spooner-blog/10-exercises-improve-vertical-jump/

Stack. (n.d.). *An 8-week training program for a higher vertical jump.* Retrieved December 8, 2024, from https://www.stack.com/a/an-8-week-training-program-for-a-higher-vertical-jump/

Zatsiorsky, V. M., & Kraemer, W. J. (2006). *Science and practice of strength training* (2nd ed.). Human Kinetics.

Zourdos, M. (2020). *Vertical jump training program: Tips to maximize power output.* Retrieved December 8, 2024, from https://simplifaster.com/articles/vertical-jump/

www.ingramcontent.com/pod-product-compliance
Lightning Source LLC
Chambersburg PA
CBHW051650250726
48653CB00007B/2583